MW01233019

SELF-HYPNOSIS FOR BEGINNERS

Lose Weight Fast with Hypnosis and Guided Meditation for Women. Learn how to Deep Sleep, Overcome Anxiety, Insomnia and Depression.

Erika Young

© Copyright 2021 - All rights reserved.

The content contained within this book may not be reproduced, duplicated or transmitted without direct written permission from the author or the publisher.

Under no circumstances will any blame or legal responsibility be held against the publisher, or author, for any damages, reparation, or monetary loss due to the information contained within this book. Either directly or indirectly.

Legal Notice: This book is copyright protected. This book is only for personal use. You cannot amend, distribute, sell, use, quote or paraphrase any part, or the content within this book, without the consent of the author or publisher.

Disclaimer Notice: Please note the information contained within this document is for educational and entertainment purposes only. All effort has been executed to present accurate, up to date, and reliable, complete information. No warranties of any kind are declared or implied. Readers acknowledge that the author is not engaging in the rendering of legal, financial, medical or professional advice. The content within this book has been derived from various sources. Please consult a licensed professional before attempting any techniques outlined in this book.

By reading this document, the reader agrees that under no circumstances is the author responsible for any losses, direct or indirect, which are incurred as a result of the use of the information contained within this document, including, but not limited to, — errors, omissions, or inaccuracies.

TABLE OF CONTENTS

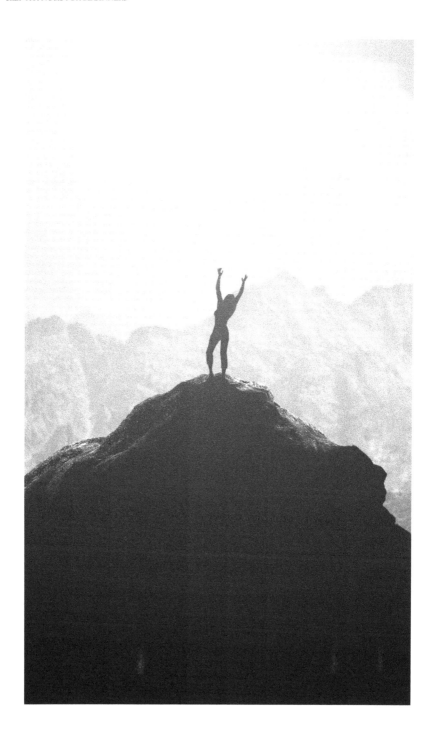

Introduction

Hypnosis for weight loss is basically using hypnosis techniques to allow you to lose weight. It is advisable that you continue a good regimen of food, followed by moderate exercise. But this will allow you to lose weight faster, and if you're a person who has cravings for things, then this will help you immensely.

It's also a part of the counseling that some people get. You'll be able to get help on your issues regarding food, and this form of hypnosis will allow you to have a better time with your cravings.

You can do this with a professional, but you can also do it on your own. It'll allow you to be in control of your life, and you'll control those bad cravings you have.

How it works is simple. When you're using hypnosis, you're in a state of absorption and concentration. You're also in a very relaxed and suggestible state, so whatever is said to you is basically taken in a literal manner.

You will use mental images to convey the meaning of the words that are said. You'll have your attention focused on that, and when your mind is in a state of concentration, you'll start to have your subconscious handle your cravings.

It's a remarkable way to keep yourself in check, and you'll be able to lose a few extra pounds while still trying to keep your body in shape. It's best if you do this with a diet and exercise routine, for it'll allow you to get through it better and achieve more results.

It's best to do this when you have a window of time ready for you to take care of this issue. You'll want at least thirty minutes of quiet time to handle these cravings, ideally an hour at most.

You will be handling some pretty heavy matters, so making sure that you're relaxed and able to come back to reality before and after the hypnosis will make it all the better.

The effectiveness varies from person to person. It will help you, and, on average, a person loses about six pounds. You might lose more, but you might not lose as much as expected. If you're trying to lose a ton of weight, this might not help.

There are other benefits of using hypnosis for weight loss. The obvious big one is that you lose weight. That's the one people will notice. You'll start to shed those pounds, and you might lose more than you expected. It won't be significant, such as like fifty pounds or more, but if you want to help your body and allow yourself the benefits of being able to control the cravings to lose weight, then this is perfect for you.

Another benefit that people don't realize is how relaxed you are. You'll actually be able to become more relaxed as a result of this. By relaxing the body, you'll be able to also reduce your blood pressure levels and even stop the risk of heart disease. Hypnosis for weight loss allows you to put yourself in a relaxed state for at least an hour, and when you wake up, you'll feel more relaxed. It can also help with bodily tissues, such as muscle aches and pains. If you want to use this to help with those issues as well, it'll definitely do the trick.

Then there are the lasting benefits of it. These are the benefits that you'll get because of the hypnosis. When you're doing this, you'll be able to tackle those parts of your subconscious that think it's okay to eat when you're stressed, or it'll tell you to eat more than necessary. Sometimes, your mind can be your own worst enemy, and this is certainly one of those times.

With hypnosis for weight loss, you'll allow yourself to handle your body in a positive manner. If you do this, you'll actually allow yourself to control your cravings and desires through the use of hypnosis. It might seem crazy, but it is possible. It's a great way to take life by the horns, and by doing this, you'll be able to allow yourself the benefit of controlling the factors in your life, such as stress or how much you eat, and turning them around to give yourself a more positive image that will benefit you in ways you've never expected before.

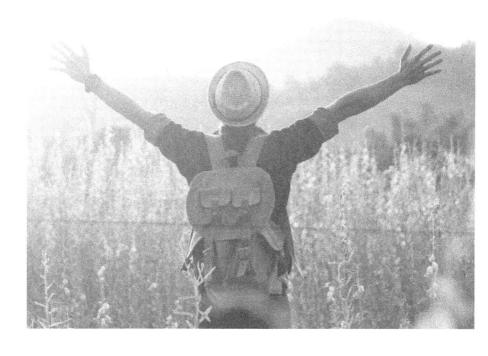

1. The Power of Repeated Words and Thoughts

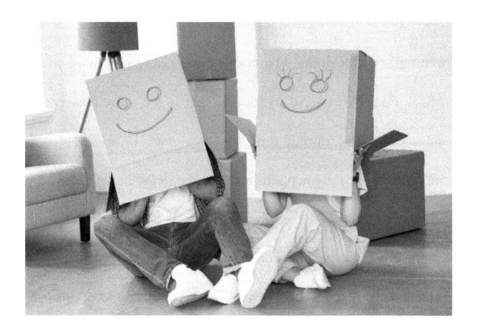

Experts estimate that an average adult experiences sixty thousand thoughts in a day. Fifty thousand of these are negative. A whopping eighty percent of our thoughts are negative and unproductive. Repetitive negative thoughts can cause illness and negative outcomes in our lives. Words have a remarkable effect on our lives. They provide us with a means to share our selves and our life experiences with others. The words we regularly use affect the experiences we have in our lives. By switching up your vocabulary, you can switch up your life.

Repetition is a powerful learning tool as it is known as the "mother" of all learning. Hypnotherapists utilize repetition wisely to pack on all aspects of hypnosis. That is the same reason that relaxes the mind during repetitive hypnosis. It is said that if something frequently happens to a desired degree or amount, you will be persuaded. That is why adverts will play consistently and on repeat because repetition is about creating a familiar pattern in abundance. When you experience something over and over again, the mind understands the phenomena causing the experience to become lodged in your memory. It is repeated so many times that it becomes convincing and to some extent, nagging. Like when a chewing gum song will not leave your mind, and you keep repeating it all day long.

Repetitive thought has made its way into our lives through many channels. Remember the Lord's Prayer? We can recite it by heart because it was pounded in us at an early age. So were nursery rhymes like "Row your boat." Repetition is present in songs, musical notes, prayers, chants, mantras, and many other forms of literary works. We assign weight and importance to our thoughts to determine which ones stay longer in our minds. Repetition is often reacted to as a social cue from a colleague. When people witness something done repetitively, they too begin to do it. That is how social media has become the plague it is.

When emotions are linked to certain things, repetition can be used as a trigger to awaken those emotions. The hypnotic triple is a hypnosis rule of thumb in some schools that states that something is suggested three times to culminate an effect. Not merely saying the words thrice, but also including the theme and any emotion that may be associated with it. The mind enjoys repetition because it is calming, and calming is always good. Therefore, reconstructing your subconscious mind to have dominant positive beliefs, thoughts, and habits, the more favorable your outlook on life will be.

Repetition and the Subconscious Mind

Your subconscious mind is impartial, unrelenting, and faithful. It does most of the sifting through all of our thoughts and relates them with our senses then communicates with the conscious mind through emotions. The subconscious mind collects your thoughts and stimuli from your environment and works on forming reactions to it. For example, you may see a particular person, perhaps your neighbor and feel dislike; you may even form a scowl. Yet, you have never exchanged three words with your neighbor. Why do you feel like this towards him/her? The information you fed your subconscious. The illusory truth effect is a phenomenon where something arbitrary becomes true because it was repeated over and over again when no one was paying any attention to it.

However, we do not know what the unconscious mind is working on because it does its works "behind the scenes." We cannot "sense" it hard at work, nor can we stop its processes. The good news then is that you can feed your mind with certain notions and ideals to elicit the emotions you have associated with them. Do not think, however, that the subconscious mind listens to reason; remember it remains an impartial participant in your everyday life. Take an example and remember when you tried to reason with an irrational phobia- of heights or tight spaces- for example. The conscious mind knows for a fact that there is nothing to fear, but you cannot help reacting in a particular way to these fears like getting sick, for example, and feeling dizzy.

Therefore, because your subconscious mind goes in the direction you command it; if you repeatedly affirm positive thoughts such as "I am beautiful," or "I can do this," you will automatically begin to develop a different attitude towards yourself. You will develop an inner outlook of your life which will gingerly propel you toward recognizing and taking advantage of the opportunities that come knocking at your door. The conscious mind can willingly train the subconscious mind and test the outcome using your life experiences. An excellent example of this is the power of autosuggestion. Have you heard of a vision board? They are ideas or fantasies that you pin up on a board that is strategically placed near the eye line. The more you repeatedly see the board, the more information you are giving the subconscious mind. After a while, check to see if there are any notable improvements in your life. For most people, it takes roughly three months to see some progress, depending on how powerful your autosuggestions are.

Affirmations and Belief

Beliefs are formed by repetitive thought that has been nourished over and over for an extended period. Affirmations are positively charged proclamations or pronouncements repeated severally through the day, every day. These words are often terse, straightforward, memorable, and repetitive. Affirmations are phrased in the present tense and they lead to belief. The most crucial element of any self-improvement process is to set an intention. Muhammud Ali once said that "It is the repetition of affirmations that cause belief, and when the beliefs become deep convictions, that is when things start to happen."

Let's say you intend to shed some weight. That being the sole goal, it is paramount that all your efforts are focused on achieving it. Therefore, affirmative statements should be in the lines of, "Shedding pounds is as easy as packing them on," "I am what I eat," "A healthy mind is a healthy body," "I feel beautiful on the outside as I do on the inside," and so on. Keep in mind that not all the words you utter will yield results. For affirmations to work, they have to be coupled with visualization and a feeling of conviction. Therefore, it is advisable to focus more on positive thoughts than negative thoughts and for a prolonged period.

Remember to use words that resonate with you. The affirmations need not be empty for you. They ought to have a close relation and meaning attached to them. The proper statements for the appropriate situation go a long way in achieving success.

You can try repeating your affirmations before you go to bed. As the brain gets ready to go on "autopilot" mode, the subconscious mind becomes more active, thereby absorbing the last bits of information for the day. Repeating affirmations before you sleep not only makes you slip into dreamland in a more confident and relaxed state but also helps to convince the mind.

You might begin to wonder why, if affirmations work, they are not used to get out of "tricky" situations. For example, if you are feeling sick, would you proceed to state, "I am cured. I am well,"? Affirmations work best with an aligned state of mind. If you believe to be well, it is more likely that you will begin to notice a decline in symptoms. If you do not believe in your affirmations, you will continue to battle through the temperature and other physical discomforts.

Finding the right words to use can be a stroll in the park; however, remembering to repeat these words, severally could present itself as a challenge. The other obstacle you might face is having two conflicting thoughts. One of them is the carefully considered affirmation, while the other is a counterproductive negation. Try the best you can to disprove the negative thoughts but do not feed them time nor energy. It will be quite challenging to believe affirmations too at the beginning. However, as time goes on, it will become easier to convince yourself. Practice makes perfect.

Affirmations seem to work because:

- The act of repeating positive statements anchors your thoughts and energy, driving you toward their fulfillment

- Affirmations program the subconscious mind, which in turn processes your reactions to circumstances.

- The more frequently you repeat the affirmations, you become more attuned with your environment. You start seeing new opportunities, and your mind opens up to new ways of fulfilling your goals

Repetition and Hypnosis

Hypnosis aims at the subconscious part of our minds to elicit lasting behavioral changes. As we have already established, repetition relaxes the mind, and when it is employed in hypnosis, the patient arrives at a state of extreme relaxation. Hypnotic suggestions can yield positive outcomes provided the intentions are set. There are two techniques used to harness the power of repetition in hypnosis.

Listen then Repeat

To bring about success during hypnosis, you must be a good listener. When someone is speaking to you, listen cautiously to both their verbal and non-verbal cues. See what both their conscious and subconscious minds are telling you. If possible, note them down.

Then say it back to them. Repeat their suggestions back to them in the language they used. When you say something in a similar tone and style, the person tends to take it as "The Gospel." Notwithstanding they feel heard and find their thoughts acceptable when they are repeated. For example, if someone says to you "I want to shed some weight to feel more like myself," you may report back to them, "You have shed some weight, and you are feeling more like yourself." Suppose you said, "You are thin, and you are feeling more like yourself." That suggestion would be utterly useless because the language used was different, therefore ineffective.

Repetitive Themes

Because themes can mean different things to different people, they become a powerful suggestive tool. Let's say a specific client always talks about one particular direction in all the meetings. Losing weight and becoming more of themselves, for instance. Take the recurrent theme and run with it. The best hypnotherapists deliver the same piece of information is a variety of ways through repetition to reinforce the principle.

You can use repetitive themes to formulate smart suggestions that are more powerful. If the subject is narrow and too specific, allow your client to broaden the topic and use the information to generalize their theme.

When appropriately applied, both techniques offer simplicity and effectiveness because hypnotherapy patients have the solutions within themselves, not to mention the brain is soothed by repetition. Therefore, the power of personal suggestion is comfortable and safe.

Using Affirmations During Self-hypnosis

It is important to reiterate that set and setting are of paramount concern. That means that it is advisable to conduct self-hypnosis in an environment where you are not likely to be disturbed- not while operating machinery or working. Let the people in your proximity know that you will be taking a nap (because hypnosis is much like falling asleep- except with heightened sensitivity) this way; you will not be interrupted.

Step 1: Write Your Script

Ensure that the text includes the beginning that is the relaxation technique. Here, you will add the repetitive sounds and if possible, visions of the ocean, if you love the ocean waves, or the sound of falling rain, or perhaps the forest. This element will relax you, and you will begin to feel physically relaxed and comfortable.

While you are in the relaxed space, repeat your affirmations about ten to fifteen times with natural deep breaths between each mantra. Continue enjoying the comfortable space you are in, taking in the smells, sights, sounds, and temperature. As you draw in all the senses from the space you are in, add to them the emotions triggered that particular "safe" space. As you start to feel, repeat the affirmations one more time. The conclusion of your script should include a dissociation between the trance state and the reality.

Step 2: Record Your Script

Talk slowly into the recording device. Slow your pace and remember your intention for doing this. The result will be more impactful if you slow your roll and allow the subconscious mind to absorb the words as you say them. The affirmations should include statements like, "I am 10-pounds lighter," "I have control over my body," and the like.

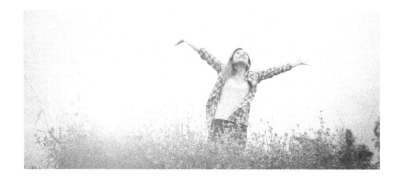

Step 3: Find a Quiet, Comfortable Space Where You Will Remain Uninterrupted for a Few Minutes

Keep in mind that when you are attempting a hypnotherapy session, the body temperature tends to fall below average. You can prepare for this using blankets or warm clothing. Put on your earpieces and listen to your recording.

Become aware of your eyelids getting heavier, and heavier as you gradually close your eyes. Remember to maintain a steady breathing motion- not too fast, not too slow. The breaths should be natural, do not struggle or pant for air. With every breath, feel yourself becoming more relaxed.

All the while keeps your mind's eye focused on the repetitive swing of the pendulum. Count slowly downwards. Start from a comfortable number, perhaps eight or ten and with each number take a deep breath into relaxation. Believe that when you finish the countdown, you will have arrived at your ideal trance state. Once you arrive, it is time to pay attention to your affirmations.

Step 4: Listen to the Recording Every Day

Commitment is key. As you listen to your affirmations, make sure to repeat them.

It is also necessary to clear your mind before attempting to get into a hypnotic state. There are several ways of clearing the mind; for example, in the advent of hypnosis, a pendulum was used to draw the attention of the mind and maintain it. The repetitive motion of the swing causes the mind to slip into a trance state. The more you repeat the process of self-hypnosis, the easier it will become for you to reach a hypnotic state, and successfully alter your life.

The law of repetition states that repetition of behavior causes it to be more potent as each suggestion acted upon creates less opposition for the following suggestions. If you are looking to change your habits, it is of uttermost importance that you are prepared to put in the work. Reprogramming the mind towards more real life-fulfilling goals can be an uphill climb because when habits form, they become harder to break and more comfortable to follow for all organs involved. However, all of that is learned in muscle memory. That is why repetition is emphasized. Meaning that because the mind is a muscle, it can be trained to take in more information, or rewrite existing knowledge. Just like the gym, it requires a commitment to see the results. As you practice repetition frequently, maintain actionable momentum on the subconscious and conscious levels of learning. Repetition is how successes are created.

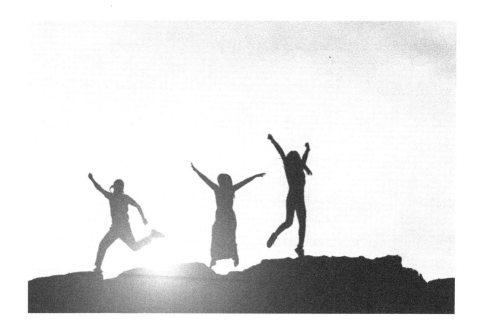

2.   Affirmation to Cut Calories

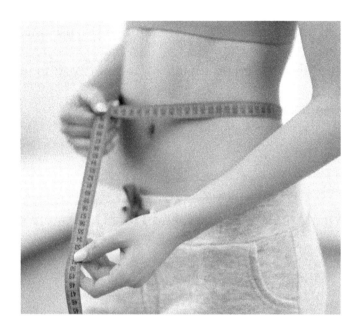

Affirmations are a wonderful tool to use alongside hypnosis to help you rewire your brain and improve your weight loss abilities. Affirmations are essentially a tool that you use to remind you of your chosen "rewiring" and to encourage your brain to opt for your newer, healthier mindset over your old unhealthy one. Using affirmations is an important part of anchoring your hypnosis efforts into your daily life, so it is important that you use them on a routine basis.

When using affirmations, it is important that you use ones that are relevant and that are going to actually support you in anchoring your chosen reality into your present reality.

What Are Affirmations, and How Do They Work?

Anytime you repeat something to yourself out loud, or in your thoughts, you are affirming something to yourself. We use affirmations on a consistent basis, whether we consciously realize it or not. For example, if you are on your weight loss journey and you repeat "I am never going to lose the weight" to yourself on a regular basis, you are affirming to yourself that you are never going to succeed with weight loss. Likewise, if you are consistently saying, "I will always be fat" or "I am never going to reach my goals" you are affirming those things to yourself, too.

When we use affirmations unintentionally, we often find ourselves using affirmations that can be hurtful and harmful to our psyche and our reality. You might find yourself locking into becoming a mental bully toward yourself as you consistently repeat things to yourself that are unkind and even downright mean. As you do this, you affirm a lower sense of self-confidence, a lack of motivation, and a commitment to a body shape and wellness journey that you do not actually want to maintain.

Affirmations, whether positive or negative, conscious, or unconscious, are always creating or reinforcing the function of your brain and mindset. Each time you repeat something to yourself, your subconscious mind hears it and strives to make it a part of your reality. This is because your subconscious mind is responsible for creating your reality and your sense of identity. It creates both around your affirmations since these are what you perceive as being your absolute truth; therefore, they create a "concrete" foundation for your reality and identity to rest on. If you want to change these two aspects of yourself and your experience, you are going to need to change what you are routinely repeating to yourself so that you are no longer creating a reality and identity rooted in negativity.

In order to change your subconscious experience, you need to consciously choose positive affirmations and repeat them on a constant basis to help you achieve the reality and identity that you truly want. This way, you are more likely to create an experience that reflects what you are looking for, rather than an experience that reflects what your conscious and subconscious mind has automatically picked up on.

The key with affirmations is that you need to understand that your brain does not care if you are creating them on purpose or not. It also does not care if you are creating healthy and positive ones or unhealthy and negative ones. All your subconscious mind cares about is what is repeated to it, and what you perceive as being your absolute truth. It is up to you and your conscious mind to recognize that negative and unhealthy affirmations will hold you back, prevent you from experiencing positive experiences in life, and result in you feeling incapable and unmotivated. Alternatively, consciously choosing healthy and positive affirmations will help you with creating a mindset that is healthier and an identity that actually serves your wellbeing on a mental, physical, emotional, and spiritual level. From there, your responsibility is to consistently repeat these affirmations to yourself until you believe them, and you begin to see them being reflected in your reality.

How Do I Pick and Use Affirmations for Weight Loss?

Choosing affirmations for your weight loss journey requires you to first understand what it is that you are looking for, and what types of positive thoughts are going to help you get there. You can start by identifying what your dream is, what you want your ideal body to look and feel like, and how you want to feel as you achieve your dream of losing weight. Once you have identified what your dream is, you need to identify what current beliefs you have around the dream that you are aspiring to achieve. For example, if you want to lose 25 pounds so that you can have a healthier weight, but you believe that it will be incredibly hard to lose that weight, then you know that your current beliefs are that losing weight is hard. You need to identify every single belief surrounding your weight loss goals and recognize which ones are negative or are limiting and preventing you from achieving your goal of losing weight.

After you have identified which of your beliefs are negative and unhelpful, you can choose affirmations that are going to help you change your beliefs. Typically, you want to choose an affirmation that is going to help you completely change that belief in the opposite direction. For example, if you think "losing weight is hard," your new affirmation could be "I lose the weight effortlessly." Even if you do not believe this new affirmation right now, the goal is to repeat it to yourself enough that it becomes a part of your identity and, inevitably, your reality. This way, you are anchoring in your hypnosis sessions, and you are effectively rewiring your brain in between sessions, too.

As you use affirmations to help you achieve weight loss, I encourage you to do so in a way that is intuitive to your experience. There is no right or wrong way to approach affirmations, as long as you are using them on a regular basis. Once you feel yourself effortlessly believing in an affirmation, you can start incorporating new affirmations into your routine so that you can continue to use your affirmations to improve your wellbeing overall. Ideally, you should always be using positive affirmations even after you have seen the changes you desire, as affirmations are a wonderful way to help naturally maintain your mental, emotional, and physical wellbeing.

What Should I Do with My Affirmations?

After you have chosen what affirmations you want to use, and which ones are going to feel best for you, you need to know what to do with them! The simplest way to use your affirmations is to pick 1-2 affirmations and repeat them to yourself on a regular basis. You can repeat them anytime you feel the need to re-affirm something to yourself, or you can repeat them continually even if they do not seem entirely relevant in the moment. The key is to make sure that you are always repeating them to yourself so that you are more likely to have success in rewiring your brain and achieving the new, healthier, and more effective beliefs that you need to improve the quality of your life.

In addition to repeating your affirmations to yourself, you can also use them in many other ways. One way that people like using affirmations is by writing them down. You can write your affirmations down on little notes and leave them around your house, or you can make a ritual out of writing your affirmations down a certain amount of times per day in a journal so that you are able to routinely work them into your day. Some people will also meditate on their affirmations, meaning that they essentially meditate and then repeat the affirmations to themselves over and over in a meditative state. If repeating your affirmation to yourself like a mantra is too challenging, you can also say your chosen affirmations to yourself on a voice recording track and then repeat them to yourself on loop while you meditate. Other people will create recordings of themselves repeating several affirmations into their voice recorder and then listening to them on loop while they work out, eat, drive to work, or otherwise engage in an activity where affirmations might be useful.

If you really want to make your affirmations effective and get the most out of them, you need to find a way to essentially bombard your brain with this new information. The more effectively you can do this, the more your subconscious brain is going to pick up on it and continue to reinforce your new neural pathways with these new affirmations. Through that, you will find yourself effortlessly and naturally believing in the new affirmations that you have chosen for yourself.

How Are Affirmations Going to Help Me Lose Weight?

Affirmations are going to help you lose weight in a few different ways. First and foremost, and probably most obvious, is the fact that affirmations are going to help you get in the mindset of weight loss. To put it simply: you cannot sit around believing nothing is going to work and expect things to work for you. You need to be able to cultivate a motivated mindset that allows you to create success. If you are unable to believe that it will come true: trust that it will not come true.

As your mindset improves, your subconscious mind is actually going to start changing other things within your body, too. For example, rather than creating desires and cravings for things that are not healthy for you, your body will begin to create desires and cravings for things that are healthy for you. It will also stop creating inner conflict around making the right choices and taking care of yourself. In fact, you may even find yourself actually falling in love with your new diet and your new exercise routine. You will also likely find yourself naturally leaning toward behaviors and habits that are healthier for you without having to try so hard to create those habits. In many cases, you might create habits that are healthy for you without even realizing that you are creating those habits. Rather than having to consciously become aware of the need for habits, and then putting in the work to create them, your body and mind will naturally begin to recognize the need for better habits and will create those habits naturally as well.

Some studies have also suggested that using affirmations will help your brain and subconscious mind actually govern your body differently, too. For example, you may be able to improve your body's ability to digest things and manage your weight naturally by using affirmations and hypnosis. In doing so, you may be able to subconsciously adjust which hormones, chemicals, and enzymes are created within your body to help with things like digestive functions, energy creation, and other weight- and health-related concerns that you may have.

Affirmations for Self-Control

Self-control is an important discipline to have, and not having it can lead to behaviors that are known for making weight loss more challenging. If you are struggling with self-control, the following affirmations will help you change any beliefs you have around self-control so that you can start approaching food, exercise, weight loss, and wellness in general with healthier beliefs.

1. I have self-control.

2. My willpower is my superpower.

3. I am in complete control of myself in this experience.

4. I make my own choices.

5. I have the power to decide.

6. I am dedicated to achieving my goals.

7. I will make the best choice for me.

8. I succeed because I have self-control.

9. I am capable of working through hardships.

10. I am dedicated to overcoming challenges.

11. My mind is strong, powerful, and disciplined.

12. I am in control of my desires.

13. My mindset is one of success.

14. I become more disciplined every day.

15. Self-discipline comes easily for me.

16. Self-control comes easily for me.

17. I achieve success because I am in control.

18. I find it easier to succeed every day.

19. I see myself as a successful, self-disciplined person.

20. Self-control comes effortlessly for me.

21. Self-control is as natural as breathing.

22. I have control over my thoughts.

23. I have control over my choices.

24. I can trust my willpower to carry me through.

25. I can tap into self-control whenever I need to.

26. My self-control is stronger than my desire.

27. I am incredibly strong with self-control.

28. I easily maintain my self-control in all situations.

29. I see things through to the end.

30. I can depend on myself to make healthy choices.

31. Healthy choices are easy for me to make.

32. It is easy for me to control my impulses.

33. Self-control is my natural state.

34. I will keep going until I reach my goal.

35. I am starting to love the feeling of self-control.

36. I see myself as a successful person.

37. I have unbreakable willpower.

38. I have excellent self-control.

39. I am a highly self-disciplined person.

40. I succeed with every goal I create.

41. I am a highly intentional person.

42. Every day, my self-control gets stronger.

43. I am becoming highly disciplined.

44. I am successful because of my self-discipline.

45. I am a strong, capable person.

46. I am dedicated to achieving my wellness goals.

47. Self-control is one of my greatest strengths.

48. I am in complete control of this situation.

49. I can do this.

50. I am self-aware and capable.

51. I can move forward with self-control and gratitude.

52. I always do what I say I am going to do.

53. I show up as my best self, and I achieve my dreams.

54. I have the willpower to make this happen.

55. I can count on myself to make the right choice.

56. I trust my strength to carry me through.

57. I am becoming stronger every day.

58. I make my choices with self-discipline.

59. I have the discipline to see this through.

60. I make my choices intentionally.

61. I am committed to my success.

Affirmations for Exercise

Exercise is necessary for healthy weight loss, but it can be challenging to commit to. Many people struggle with motivating themselves to exercise, or to exercise enough, to take proper care of their body. If you are struggling with exercising, these affirmations will help motivate you to work out or motivate you to finish your workout on a high note.

1. I am so excited to exercise.

2. I love moving my body.

3. I am focused and ready to exercise.

4. I am showing up at 100%.

5. Today, I will have an excellent workout.

6. I have the courage to see this workout through.

7. My body is becoming stronger every day.

8. I love exercising.

9. Exercising is fun and exciting.

10. I love becoming the best version of myself.

11. Exercising is one of my favorite activities.

12. Exercising makes me feel happy and healthy.

13. I have a strong body and mind.

14. I am confident about my ability to see this through.

15. I can feel myself becoming stronger.

16. I can feel myself becoming leaner.

17. My body is getting healthier every single day.

18. I am transforming my body every day.

19. I am creating the body I have always wanted.

20. Every day I am losing weight.

21. I am getting thinner every single day.

22. Each day I get closer to my ideal weight.

23. I am motivated to take care of my body.

24. I am excited to lose weight in a healthy, natural way.

25. My body is capable of being healthy.

26. I love how flexible my body is becoming.

27. Maintaining my ideal weight is as easy as breathing.

28. My weight is dropping quickly and in a healthy way.

29. I am dedicated to having a stronger body.

30. I feel myself getting stronger every single day.

31. My body deserves a healthy workout.

32. I love creating my dream body.

33. Having a strong body is important to me.

34. I am motivated to reach my fitness goals.

35. I am determined to have a healthier body.

36. I am so proud of myself for my growth.

37. I am strong and motivated.

38. I am committed to having a healthier body.

39. I easily become motivated to exercise.

40. I am capable of having a healthier body.

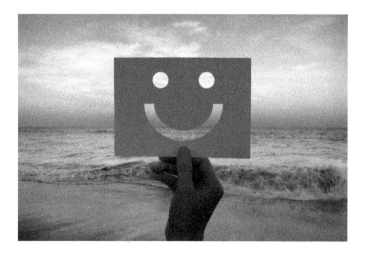

3. Low of Attraction

Your thoughts can be used for good or bad without even realizing it. Unfortunately, most of what we see and hear today is negative. News, media, music, coworkers, and even family members can spread negative thoughts with no direct intention. When our minds are taking in negative information, that becomes our thoughts and our thoughts become our actions.

Scientists tell us that our thoughts generate unique frequencies that attract back to us like frequencies. This is known as the Law of Attraction. This universal law states that we generate the things, events, and people that appear in our lives. Our thoughts, feelings, words, and actions produce energies (unique frequency) that attract like energies. Negative energies attract negative energies and positive energies attract positive energies.

This means nothing happens in our lives by coincidence. You attract everything into your life, everything that happens to you, through your thoughts, feelings, words, and actions. Notice that this chain of events begins with your thoughts. Knowing this will make it easier to understand why having negative thoughts of depression, anger, hatred, greed, or selfishness to name a few, can bring you more of the same.

By learning to directly control your thoughts, you are able to block out negative energies. This can be accomplished by thinking only positive thoughts. Positive thinking is a theory that many ancient masters and philosophers have used throughout history.

Successful men and women have used positive thinking to inspire thousands. Many teachers and motivational speakers today use the power of positive thinking to help change people's lives for the better. This positive thinking technique is easier said than done however.

To think positively you have to concentrate on your thoughts, especially at first. The minute your subconscious mind takes over, it can fall back into old habits of negative thinking. Practicing to think positive all day long will take some effort considering we have 35-48 thoughts per minute. Being persistent in regard to thinking positively will eventually become a habit and a new way of life.

You will start to notice good things happening to you. You'll notice things seem to fall into place and go your way. Do not dismiss this phenomenon as a mere coincidence. It is great powers at work. The more evidence you obtain that it's working, the easier it will become to master. Before you know it, you'll be living the life you've always dreamed of. A life of success and happiness anyone would appreciate.

Most people underestimate the power of their thoughts. They think that thought is nothing, that thoughts are not things, and therefore that they cannot affect reality. Science has already shown that this is not true, our ways of thinking determine most of the things that happen to us, we just don't realize it. You can easily see it paying attention to the little everyday things, for example how a thought, an emotion or a state of mind instantly influence your physiology and your body.

Think about when you are afraid; the thought of something that scares you can increase sweating, accelerate the heartbeat and breathing. In the same way, even the less important sensations for survival, like a positive emotion, can have real physical effects.

Think for example when you listen to a song that you like or that gives you intense emotions, it is not a mere sensation that stops only in the mind, it spreads like a wave in the whole body, some people, for example, get goosebumps ... This means that thought has had a physical, real and tangible effect on their body and their physiology.

Thoughts have the power not only directly on you, but they shape the reality in which you live. A positive thought attracts positive things and shifts your focus to positive events, it is a bit like when you are driving and you are late, you will find many more red lights on your path, in reality you are the one who puts the focus on the obstacles, so you notice much more negative things and you feel therefore unlucky, which increases your attention even more in noticing negative things, thus creating a destructive spiral. Remember, anything you focus on, will grow.

Then, the regular and constant repetition over time of positive affirmations can reprogram our brain on a positive mindset, and creates a virtuous circle in which we begin to notice more positive things and consequently leads us to receive them in greater quantity, creating an infinite loop of gratitude and attraction of the good.

Your faith and your love are energy, which, by interacting with the energy of the universe, will attract to you everything you want strongly.

The affirmations you are about to hear, if repeated a sufficient number of times, will become rooted in your unconscious and will replace the negative paradigms you may have developed from your childhood until today. This process will change the lenses through which you look at the world and your life will turn into something wonderful and unique, making you grateful and able to appreciate all the things you have and will attract.

The Law of Attraction is not a new concept. It's always been around and it's constantly working, whether you believe in it or not. You can't get better at using the Law of Attraction because you're already using it. It already does work perfectly, 100% of the time. Practical Law of Attraction helps you get better at getting into alignment with the manifesting conditions, so you can manifest your heart's desire.

Perhaps you've heard it defined as "ask, believe, and achieve," or some other 3-step process.

These featured steps are important elements to manifesting. However, it goes way deeper than that. What about action? When they say "believe," are they saying consciously or unconsciously?

Certainly, if you focus on those three steps, it's possible you might get results. However, if you are getting results focusing on only those three steps, then it's because you are unconsciously also applying some unmentioned steps.

If you haven't been getting results, then you'll understand why as we go through the manifesting conditions.

Here's How I Define Law of Attraction:

"Law of Attraction is when the manifesting conditions and personal qualities are developed and come into alignment simultaneously."

It's an impersonal law. It's unbiased. In other words, it doesn't matter if what you think, imagine, feel, or believe is something you fear or something you desire, the law works the same exact way—always. It simply manifests whatever you are in alignment with.

Law of Attraction is not a quick fix. It is a way of life.

It's not a step by step formula or process, because you are starting "the process" from where you are right now, your own unique set of circumstances.

As you explore each of the manifesting conditions, you will gain a better understanding of how you have created the life situation, you're in now. You'll also learn the ways to stop creating more unwanted circumstances, and ultimately create a life you truly love.

How did Law of Attraction Originate?

The New Thought movement grew out of the teachings of Phineas Quimby in the early 19th Century. Early in his life, Quimby was diagnosed with tuberculosis. Unfortunately, medicinal treatment wasn't working.

In 1838, Quimby began studying Mesmerism. He became aware of the mental and placebo effect of the mind over the body when prescribed medicines of no physical value cured patients of diseases. From there, Phineas Quimby developed theories of mentally aided healing

It wasn't until 1877 that the term "Law of Attraction" first appeared in print, in a book which discusses esoteric mysteries of ancient theosophy, called Isis Unveiled, written by the Russian occultist, Helena Blavatsky, where she alluded to an attractive power existing between elements of spirit.

However, there have been many references even before the term was used, that describe what we understand today.

Gautama Buddha, (who lived between 563 BC - 480 BC): said "What we are today comes from our thoughts of yesterday, and our present thoughts build our life of tomorrow: Our life is the creation of our mind."

Empedocles (490 BC), an early Greek philosopher, hypothesized something called Love (philia) to explain the attraction of different forms of matter.

Plato alleged as early as (391 BC): "Like tends towards like."

The Bible has many statements suggesting the power of having faith and asking for what you want, such as: "Ask, and it shall be given you; seek, and ye shall find; knock and it shall be opened unto you."

By the 20th Century, a surge in interest in the subject led to many books being written about it, including:

The Science of Getting Rich (1910) by Wallace D. Wattles

The Master Key System (1912) Charles Haanel

How to Win Friends and Influence People (1936) Dale Carnegie

Think and Grow Rich (1937) Napoleon Hill

The Power of Positive Thinking (1952) Norman Vincent Peale

The Power of Your Subconscious Mind (1962) Joseph Murphy

Creative Visualization (1978) Shakti Gawain

You Can Heal Your Life (1980) Louise Hay

Law of Intention and Desire (1994) Deepak Chopra

How to Get What You Really, Really, Really, Really Want (1998) Wayne Dyer, public television special

The Secret (2006): The concept of the Law of Attraction gained a lot of renewed exposure with the release of the film and book written by Rhonda Byrne.

Since then, Law of Attraction became a bit more well-known. However, since the film represents the topic in a very basic manner with an inadequate basis for real-world application it contributes to some skepticism.

Things that Aren't True

Myth #1: The Law of Attraction Isn't True

It always surprises me how many bright, intelligent people there are who learn about Law of Attraction and flippantly write it off as nonsense. The only issue with Law of Attraction is one of misunderstanding of what it is and how it works.

Before you dismiss the Law of Attraction, ask yourself this: Would aligning your thoughts, feelings, beliefs, and behaviors with what you want help you or hinder you?

Here's the thing, a belief in the Law of Attraction is a belief in your ability to have control over deliberately creating your reality and manifesting whatever you desire.

The idea you have a say in how your life is going infuriates some people. I can only assume this is because they are receiving some counter intentions by remaining stuck in a belief system that supports them in maintaining a victim mentality.

If you are of the opinion that what you think and feel has no bearing on your reality, you will not be able to attract results that you desire.

The mind is set up in such a way that it favors information that conforms to your existing beliefs and discounts evidence that does not.

Remember, the Law of Attraction is always working. How it works for you is up to you.

Myth #2: The Law of Attraction Is Like a Genie Granting Your Every Wish

This is the myth which continues to perpetuate Myth #1, that it doesn't work. Since Law of Attraction does not actually work like a genie, those who go into it thinking all they need to do is make a wish and a magic genie will miraculously appear and grant their heart's desire are setting themselves up for disillusionment.

Approaching Law of Attraction, coming from this idea you can think yourself into receiving high-ticket items, like cars, dream homes, and lottery winnings, and change your life overnight, is unhealthy. It is the very reason why critics, skepticism, and misunderstanding about this Law exist.

While it's possible to achieve what you desire, it's going to require much more than thinking. It takes diligent effort to grow yourself into the person who is in alignment with your true desires.

Law of Attraction is common sense. It's a set of practical conditions the most successful people are naturally in alignment with. You need to have a clear desire and intention. Focus is required. You also need to be intentionally taking actions toward achieving what you want to create.

The more you align yourself with these conditions, the more the universal creative energy corresponds by sending you new ideas, intuitive messages, opportunities, helpful people, and other resources.

Myth #3: When Bad Stuff Happens, it is All Your Fault

No one knows exactly why catastrophic, horrible events happen to innocent, good, and well-intentioned people.

Some Law of Attraction advocates go too far and say you are responsible for every bad thing that's ever happened to you. There are no good answers to why terrible events happen to good people. I'm talking about the likes of getting raped, having your home burn down to the ground, or learning that you or a loved-one has been diagnosed with a terminal illness.

You certainly have every right to feel and process all the emotions you undergo when you experience a devastating loss or tragedy. One reason people remain stuck from moving on is they did not process their feelings. You can only heal what you feel.

The Law of Attraction is not about blaming you for everything that's ever happened to you in your life. Understand that sometimes bad things happen, like losing your job, going through a bad break-up, or not getting approved for your loan. Often enough, you can look back on those situations and see something better happened as a result, and it never would have happened had the bad thing never occurred.

What if, when bad things happened, you were to remain open to discovering how the event might play into a much grander, more intelligent plan that the universe has in store for you?

Here are a few other theories about why negative things might happen and how to deal with them when they do.

- The truth is, sometimes we do attract scenarios to ourselves by having fears about those things happening. Negative thoughts and energies do attract negative.

- If you believe in the concept that your soul has lived lives before this one, then you may be experiencing karma that originated several lifetimes ago.

- Again, if you believe in this idea that we have many lives and we create our lesson plans between lives, sometimes we orchestrate events we need to experience in this life for our soul to advance.

- It's completely random and we just don't have control over everything that happens to us. But we do have complete control over how we allow it to affect us as we navigate through our future.

The bottom line is, regardless of which scenario you subscribe to, it's tiresome and painful to try and pinpoint exactly why things happen to us. When life becomes difficult and painful, you have two options. 1) You can accept what happened; or 2) you can suffer.

Acceptance does not mean you are making the situation right or you like or want what happened. It simply means you have accepted the idea that no matter how much you dwell on it, you are not going to change what happened. Acceptance is a way of letting it go so you can make room for better things to happen.

One of the laws of nature is change or impermanence. The one constant is change. Everything and everyone will eventually die.

Make peace with the past. Accept it. Forgive it. Live in the present. Whatever happened, happened. Life is not always fair. If you are always focusing on how things were, and the injustice you feel, then you will continue to re-create your future from that state. No matter how bad it was, it is not happening now. It only exists in your memory. You do not have to let it control your thoughts, emotions, or bring it into your future.

Focus on what you have control over, which is how you choose to experience this present moment. Whatever you are focusing on, feeling, and imagining right now is what's creating your future.

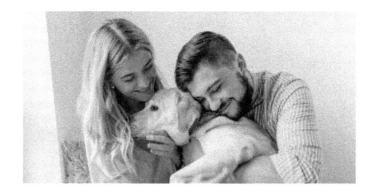

The Laws

Universal Laws

Universal Laws are guidelines that help us understand the rules we are playing by.

Everything in the world is made of energy and we are all connected with that energy.

Our thoughts, feelings, words, and actions are all forms of energy and is what creates our reality.

What's exciting about that is since our thoughts, feelings, words, and actions create the world around us, we have the power to create a world of peace, harmony, and abundance.

I've chosen to share just a few of those laws to help you understand how that is all possible.

The Law of Abundance

The Law of Abundance states that we live in an abundant universe. There is plenty of everything, including love, money, and all the necessities for everyone.

The key to having abundance is alignment with the conditions for manifesting it.

You likely grew up hearing things like "there are starving children in Africa, so you need to eat every last bite of food that is on your plate." Or "money doesn't grow on trees."

The truth is, there is abundance in the world. It is all around you. It's about what you are choosing to focus on. We don't have any issues with scarcity in the world, even when it comes to those starving children. The planet produces enough food. Hunger is not a problem caused by nature. Hunger is caused by lack of efficiency and politics.

I am illustrating how it does not serve any of us well to confuse issues like hunger, not to be ignored, with scarcity.

The Abundance Mindset

How you view the world can affect the opportunities you see, your beliefs, and ultimately your results. You can choose to see the world as a place of abundance or a place of scarcity.

An abundance mindset is hopeful, positive, and expects the best. It is also more altruistic, since you believe you'll receive what you need. It frees you up to do more for others.

A scarcity mindset, on the other hand, leads to negativity and selfishness. You feel the need to look out for yourself, even at the expense of others.

Abundance Mindset	Scarcity Mindset
There is plenty to go around. Everyone can win.	There is a limited supply of everything, and someone else must lose for you to win.
Life is easier. You believe anything is possible. Expect the best and things eventually go your way.	Life is difficult. Success is hard. You expect the worst and that's how it turns out.
Opportunities are easier to spot.	Opportunities are scarce, and you struggle to find them.

You take more risks. The bigger the risk, the bigger the reward.	You play it safe. You're afraid to lose.
You are more relaxed. You enjoy life because all your needs are met.	You live in fear and pessimism. You must fight the world to get what you want and need.

Which view do you normally see the world through? Abundance or scarcity?

One way to begin feeling the abundance, which may seem counter intuitive, is by giving more. Whatever resource you feel you lack, give that.

It feels good to give and it tricks you into believing you have plenty, which changes your energy and puts you into the flow of abundance.

How to Move from Scarcity to Abundance

1. Focus on what you already have. When you see that you already have enough, you feel abundant and are likely to attract more to you.

2. Avoid people that complain a lot. Complainers have a scarcity mindset. You're more susceptible to others' mindsets than you think. Spend time with positive people who have the mindset you want.

3. Visualize an abundant future. Instead of worrying about what you don't have, allow yourself to dream about what you want to achieve in the future.

4. Keep a positive journal. List the things in your life you feel grateful for. Be sure to mention all the people in your life. You probably have a home, a job, a car, family, friends, and so on. That's a good place to start.

5. Be generous. Demonstrate to yourself there is enough for everyone by sharing what you have, including time. The more you share, the more others want to reciprocate.

An abundance mindset won't magically put you into a Mercedes or add a few zeros to your bank account overnight. However, an abundance mindset will allow you to move forward with confidence as you take the necessary steps to make positive changes in your life.

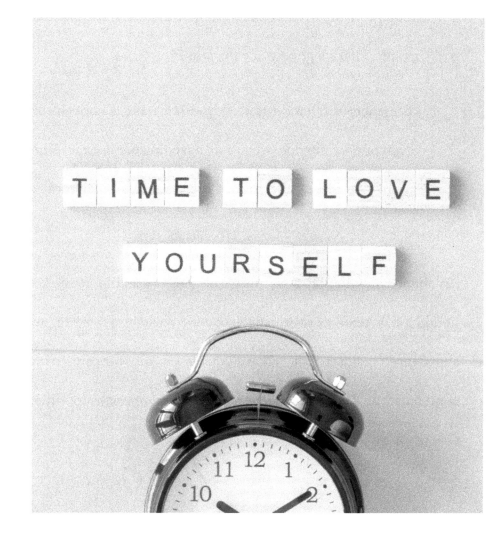

Conclusions

The key to success lies in resolving the mental imbalance so that those affected can find their inner balance and lose weight in a healthy way.

Eating disorders are often an expression of a mental imbalance. The lack of inner balance leads to blockages that prevent normal eating behavior. Practical tips and well-intentioned advice on losing weight are often ineffective because they only address awareness.

Likewise, efforts made by those concerned to eat normally and lose weight associated with conscious effort often do not lead to success. Yes, sometimes these forced efforts to lose weight actually do the opposite.

Hypnosis is a temporary state of more acute concentration. It is a totally natural state of consciousness. We constantly pass in our life from one state of concentration to another. Therefore, hypnosis is totally familiar to us because of our daily experiences.

An effective and permanent change in eating behavior is most likely to succeed if the therapy starts at the subconscious level. So, the high success rate of hypnotherapy depends on losing weight together with the fact that it is possible to communicate directly with the subconscious.

In hypnotherapy, the first step is to uncover the causes of obesity in the subconscious of a person.

Blockages that have manifested in the subconscious can be resolved in the hypnotic trance. By the way, no deep trance is required for this.

A pleasantly relaxed, light state of trance is enough to work successfully. If the blockages acquired during childhood, adolescence or even in adulthood can be successfully resolved, the eating disorder can also be overcome so that you can lose weight on your wellbeing.

If you have been eating junk food all your life or been a chronic dieter your body needs to recover.

If you have never dieted and are thinking of going on a diet, I hope that this will have put you wise about the pitfalls and dangers. In short, don't go down the road of dieting, it is full of potholes.

This way of eating will be a transition!

An end to dieting, and then finding the best way of eating and the beginning of a healthy new you.

Make this a commitment for life and not just another diet. You can have the odd treat, and even a glass of red wine sometimes with your meal.

But let the treat be just that, a treat! Not something that you are in the habit of doing all the time.

When you are eating out, ignore the jibes from friends. They will soon get used to your new and healthy way of eating, and may even follow you.

Use expressions such as "I don't eat that" rather than the disempowering "I can't eat that." This will let you keep your own power and not give it away to anybody else. "Don't" implies that YOU are in control. "Can't" implies that someone else's rules are controlling you.

Learn to cook. It is fun and you will be surprised at the concoctions that you can come up with using basic ingredients and adding spices and herbs.

Changing your thinking

Changing the way that you think can make a huge difference in your weight management. There are beliefs that we all carry around with us from childhood.

Many of them are necessary, such as cleaning your teeth because if you don't they will decay. Or wash your hands before eating and after using the bathroom, because of germs. These are just two very simple habits and beliefs. There are other more complicated ones that are passed down through families, or from parents to children, such as the type of manners we may have, or religious beliefs. But for now let's just keep it simple.

One belief that may be around is that if your parents were fat, so you will be too. You may have heard that this is genetic, or it's in the genes. But there is now a relatively new science known as epigenetics, and this is proving that although we may carry certain dispositions in our genes for illness or conditions, we can control the outcome with our environment.

For example if someone dies of lung cancer and has been a heavy smoker, their offspring can lessen their chances of getting it by not smoking.

SELF-HYPNOSIS FOR BEGINNERS

We also need to be aware of how we think in any given moment. One scenario often cited to me is people's work environment. I hear a lot about the struggle that office workers have when fellow colleagues insist on bringing in cakes for a birthday. The person who chooses not to include cake in their diet, often struggles with this, as they don't want to appear to be different and unsociable, or they feel left out.

Let's look at this a bit closer. There you are sitting at your desk and the doughnuts have arrived. Everyone is joining in and you have to make a choice.

I will cover briefly here something called resistance. There is a saying "What resists, persists" and this is true. Let's explore this a little further.

Imagine that it is the first time this has happened since you changed your way of eating, you can simply say "No thank you, I wish you a really happy day, but I am not eating that sort of food anymore". I t is not a good idea to say that you are on a diet! That is like putting a red rag in front of a bull. Our society seems to hate people saying that they are on a diet. But the idea of watching our health is more appealing.

Be warned though, you will get some remark, but stick to your new principles. Because if you don't, then next time it will be even harder. Once they get the message the first time, as each time comes around, they will become familiar with the idea.

Another way to avoid the resistance though is to just accept the situation for what it is. Have just a little piece. But promise yourself that it will indeed be the one piece.

That way there is nothing to resist. This will help you to become aware of your ability to make choices and changes.

You are in control, and just because a certain food may have affected you in the past, you can change the story, and tell yourself that any weakness from the past, does not have to affect me now.

This can be quite a challenge for some people, and some life coaching or mentoring may be useful.

By this little exercise you will have learnt to change your thinking from "I'll just have one this time" to "I like eating this way and I am not going to let a moment's weakness or embarrassment spoil it"

Think about other occasions when we say, "No", and there does not seem to be a problem. Such as not having a drink because you are driving. On a parallel with that, isn't your health just as important and not having a cake because of it?

Using positive affirmations on a daily basis can be an incredibly persuasive method for attracting health, healing, and happiness into each day of your life.

Remember, as you start each day, it's up to you to decide if it's going to be a positive one.

Everyone has to cope with the onslaught of daily life, and tackle their own personal issues, in areas such as self-esteem, fears, and disappointments.

However, by using positive affirmations, you can choose to approach life with a more positive attitude, be open to new opportunities, and expect good things to be attracted effortlessly into your world.

Throughout this, we've looked at what, why and how to use positive affirmations to gain personal strength, and to help us feel happy, healthy, and healed.

We've explored how to:

- Focus on what you really want.

- Use positive, uplifting, empowering words.

- Re-condition your subconscious, away from toxic thoughts.

- Understand why affirmations can fail.

- Identify the most beneficial affirmations for you.

- Correctly use the most effective techniques.

- Create believable statements that feel really good.

- Show gratitude for the positive changes in your life.

- Expect good things.

Positive affirmations, when used correctly, can offer a simple, fast and effective method for delivering long lasting change into your life. When you start to believe you are better, both physically and mentally, you will start to receive corresponding physical benefits to your health. W

hen you feel more positive, you enable yourself to cope better with stress, to be more resilient to problems, and to fight off common ailments, thanks to an improved immune system.

Additionally, when you experience positive feelings, either through your engagement of affirmation techniques, or as a result of moving closer to your desired outcome, you will start to see more and more possibilities.

As you experience greater levels of emotions, such as contentment, happiness, excitement, joy, and hope, you'll open yourself up to new opportunities, and ways in which you can experience even more of the positive things in life.

The conscious use of positive affirmations helps to bring about lasting, positive change by creating new affirming beliefs, deep in your subconscious.

The consistent use of positive affirmations can be a major component in letting go of negative beliefs.

They can be used effectively to replace negative self-talk, which, when left unresolved, can have a detrimental effect on both our emotional and physical health, along with our ability to progress in any meaningful manner.

SELF-HYPNOSIS FOR BEGINNERS

"Believing in negative thoughts is the single greatest obstruction to success."~ Charles F. Glassman

There are certain fundamental aspects you need to follow when you embark on a journey of affirmations. Get these right, and your personal affirmation statements will work amazing well:

Trust	Know in your heart that they will work for you
Expectation	Expect a great outcome
Belief	Create believable personal statements
Power	Use your personal powers, and take action

Value	Be true to yourself and your purpose
Attention	Give intense focus to what you really want
Gratitude	Give daily thanks

Pay attention to these hugely important aspects, as they help fuel the transformations you seek. Understand that each point above brings its own unique benefits, allowing you to continually attract more of what you want into your life.

The art of positive affirmation needs to be practiced, and honed, and practiced, to become a perfect fit for your own purposes.

Although affirmations do not necessarily offer a quick fix, they do offer a powerful solution to create positive, lasting change. The creation of well crafted, affirming personal statements, can help recondition our thoughts and beliefs, allowing us to feel good about ourselves in so many different ways. As they work deeply at the subconscious level to affect change in both your beliefs and attitudes, they can be a driving force for delivering change exactly where you want it.

CPSIA information can be obtained
at www.ICGtesting.com
Printed in the USA
BVHW050908070421
604337BV00006B/972